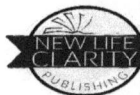

My Simple

Guide

to Healthy Eating

Written by:
Amara Janke

About the Author

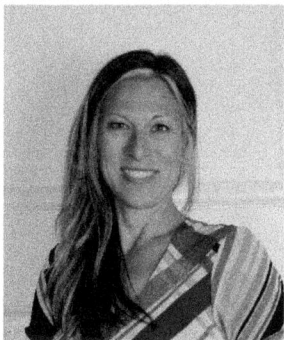

My name is Amara, I'm a single mom of two amazing little kiddos. I share two passions, being a mom and living a fit and healthy lifestyle. I first got certified as a Personal Trainer when I was 19 years old. I started going to the gym and didn't have experience so I decided to learn. I started studying nutrition at that time as well, reading every magazine and book I could about health and fitness, and taking college nutrition courses. I have lived a healthy lifestyle ever since. I love going to the gym, lifting weights, running and eating healthy. It wasn't long after that when I went to college to become a social worker. I worked in the field for 5 years but in 2009 I decided to do what I am passionate about. That was the beginning of my next adventure as I opened my business Team Crazy Fit. My company is a fitness company where I offer online and in-person personal training and meal plans. Opening my own business has been one of the most rewarding decisions of my life. I am able to do what I love daily and really help others along the way. I love to serve and truly believe, "the more you give, the more you will receive."

I am now able to share my knowledge and expertise with others to help them live healthier lifestyles. Living a healthier lifestyle isn't just about "looking good in a swimsuit", it is about being able to chase your kids around, living longer and healthier lives, feeling good about yourself. Living healthy means feeling good about yourself and increasing your energy, truly being able to really enjoy life.

Acknowledgements

I want to give a special thank you to my older sister, Carissa for all of her love and support in creating this book. Carissa was the first person to read it, re-read it, and praise me for it. She is my rock and biggest supporter.

I also want to thank all of my friends, clients, and fitness professionals who took the time to read this and give me feedback before I sent it to the publisher, supporting me in my fitness journey: Shae Bitton, Suzette Jackson, Ryan Flint, Ed Kinsey and Tyler Alexander.

I also want to thank my ex-husband Shawn Janke. He pushed me to start my fitness company, Team Crazy Fit, in 2009. He has always been supportive and believed in me.

Thank you to my wonderful family for all their love and support.

Dedication

I dedicate this book to my beautiful Children. You inspire me to be a better person every day!

Preface

My biggest goal for this book is to teach people how to eat healthy! This is truly a course I feel should be taught in school, along with how to budget money, set goals and the law of attraction.

But for this book, I am going to focus on teaching you how to make better eating choices.

I am extremely passionate about health and fitness. I first got certified as a trainer when I was 17 years old, because I wanted the knowledge of how to work out and be healthy.

My kids did not eat any sugar until their second birthday (besides natural sugars found in fruits). My son never had a vanilla wafer until he started pre-school and it was the snack for the day. It's a pretty funny story! He came home and tried to explain the snack he had. He said it was the best thing he had ever had! I called his teacher who laughed and said it was a vanilla wafer. She said he really did love them and kept asking for more! My kids were three and six before they had their first jelly bean. They came home after trying one and were so excited to tell me about them and how good they were! My kids don't eat at McDonald's, and have never had a hotdog. I know you all are thinking I'm totally crazy, but good health is so important to me! I do allow my kids to have cake at parties, or a treat if everyone else is having one. We do make cookies or stop for ice cream occasionally. Having treats and sugar is something special for them, and they thoroughly enjoy them, especially my daughter! There is balance in everything!

With that being said I also really want to point out that although I know I have a lot of control over what my kids eat now, there will be days in the future when I will not! So it's so important not to just feed our children healthy foods, but educate them on healthy foods. My son was offered a hotdog at a bbq and he told them, "No thank you, hotdogs are made out of pig butts and all the other parts of the big no one wants to eat." Educate them, empower them to make healthier choices. Explain to them what sugars do to your body, and what healthy foods do. I explain this to my 4 and 6-year-old like this; "eating junk food, sugar, cookies, candy, chips etc. fills our bodies up, and then we don't have room for the healthy foods our body needs. Like dairy products to build strong bones, proteins to build muscle, etc.". (I go over all this in the book). I also talk to them while we are eating what they are eating, "chicken is a protein, protein helps build muscle. Lettuce is a veggie it gives your body needed vitamins and minerals."

My goal for this book isn't to be the thickest, longest book you have ever read, or to give you a degree in nutrition. I just want to give you some simple advice on how to eat healthier and teach you and your children how to make healthier food choices. Obesity is an ongoing problem. Besides all the health issues that come with obesity and unhealthy eating, you and your children's self-esteem will suffer from being overweight. It breaks my heart to see children being teased at school because of their weight and teens who let others take advantage of them because of their low self-body image. My goal is to bring more awareness to this topic, and truly make you see it is easy to do once you get started. Meal prepping and eating foods without mayonnaise or butter is a big adjustment at first, but after a few weeks you will enjoy your food without it just as much as you did with it.

I also want to note that I am not a certified nutritionist; however, have been studying nutrition for twenty years. I am not here to write big words and sound extra smart. I just want this to be an easy guide for you follow to help you make better health choices for you and your kids.

Eating is the biggest part of your success in meeting your health and fitness goals; however, being active and working out has its important place as well. I highly recommend you finding at least 30 minutes a day to move; go for a walk, take the stairs, dance, mow the yard, just be active for at least 30 minutes a day. If you need a workout plan, please send me an email. I would love to get you a plan to help you meet your goals! Now please remember while reading this book, there are exceptions to many things. If your doctor has you doing something different than I recommend, please consult with them before making any changes. Also please keep in mind, this book is written for adults, although some of it may also pertain to children, which I will note.

When I asked people what they wanted most out of this book, I got a lot of people saying simple meal ideas, which I have included. To be honest my family eats a lot of the same foods during the week. It is easier for me to cook a big batch of chicken and eat it for the next four days than it is to cook every night. I know it can get boring to eat the same thing every day. If you want to mix it up, you can try cooking your chicken differently: in the oven, on the stove, on the barbeque, or in the crockpot or Instant pot. You can also use different seasonings to make it taste different. You have to decide what's best for your family- if you prefer the same stuff every night or if you want to make a warm dinner every night. No option is wrong, it's just what works for you and your family.

I try to look at food as a source that fuels our bodies, and that's it! Food shouldn't be companionship, a friend, a counselor, or a reward. Not that I have never used it to help me with my emotions, because I have! But if you can change your view about it to, "it's just a fuel your body needs to function". When you change the way you look at food, you will change your relationship with it. Food should not control you, it should fuel you. Food was designed in the beginning as a means to keep you alive. Your body needs certain foods and nutrients to work properly and be healthy. I can't stress this enough: try not to find too much pleasure in food, because that's not its purpose. Remind yourself you need food to survive and that is its purpose! Feeling down? Call a friend. Bored? Go for a walk. Don't use food to serve your emotions. Repeat with me, "Food is a fuel that keeps my body alive." That's it! Think of your body like a car. A car needs gas to drive, your body needs healthy food to drive. Eating clean and healthy doesn't need to be hard. It's really very simple, pick healthy foods, and eat them at the most efficient times. When you look at food in this way, it's easier to figure out what your body needs versus what your emotions want.

One last thing to add before we really dive in! YOU CAN'T OUT EAT A BAD DIET! This is such an AH-HA moment for people! Most people think, "I went to the gym for an hour today, so I can eat whatever I want now." Here's the truth. Today I ran 4.5 miles outside pushing a stroller, and according to my apple watch I burned 447 total calories. That same day I also did a 35 min ab and leg workout, and burned 143 total calories. Great job for me right?! But here's the thing, that's a total of 590 calories. Guess how many calories are in a *slice of pizza, Starbucks, McDonald's hamburger, or a can of Coke?* On average a piece of pizza has 285 calories (for 1 slice of a 14-inch pizza), a McDonald's hamburger has 250 calories, a Starbucks Java Chip Frappuccino has 220 calories, and a can of Coke has 150 calories. As you can see, food adds up quick!! If I had 2 slices of pizza in one meal, I would have eaten more calories in that meal than I burned in my 80 minutes of working out!! So trust me when I say you can't out train a bad diet. Working out is so important, but eating healthy is a must to achieve a healthy goal weight.

You've already made the first step to a healthier lifestyle, by purchasing this book. I know you can do! Start small, pick one thing your will incorporate and then once that's a habit incorporate another. Remember there will be days that you struggle and mess up, and that's ok! Even I knowing all that I know struggle some days! Even though I eat too much cake sometimes, or eat the whole bag of cookies because I already messed up so why not just eat the whole bag!?!? But that's the good thing about life, you can wake up the next day and try again. It's what you do 80% of the time, not ALL the time!! Keep your head up, continue to believe in yourself, and one step at a time make some healthier choices!!

Table of Contents

CHAPTER 1

Your Metabolism

So where to start?

Let's start with your metabolism. Your metabolism is what burns calories during the time you are not working out. In order to keep your metabolism working for you, you should eat every 2-4 hours.

I'm going to break this down really simple for you. These are not exact numbers, but it will help you understand why you need to eat more frequent, smaller meals. The only way to turn on your metabolism is by eating or working out. For easy math, I am going to say your body can only burn through 200 calories at a time (now like I said above, these are not real numbers just numbers I am using to illustrate this to you). Let's say you wake up and you eat a 200 calorie meal. By eating, you kick start your metabolism and turn it on. Your body effectively burns through those 200 calories, and is about to start slowing down. At this point, you eat again, another 200 calorie meal. You continue to do this every 2-3 hours. You eat 200 calories, your body burns it, you eat again, and your body burns it. This makes your metabolism work for you ALL day long!

Now here's another scenario. You wake up and skip breakfast, therefore your metabolism never turns on. You wait until lunch and by then, you are starving so you eat a 600 calorie lunch. Given the number above we are saying your body can only burn through 200 calories at a time, so the extra 400 are stored as fat. Now you don't eat again until dinner where you again eat 600 calories. You burn 200 of those calories and store the remaining 400 as fat. Now I know that probably 60-70% of people fall into this category of skipping meals then overeating, but as you can see this is not helping you reach your goals!!! With that being said, your body will also go into starvation mode when meals are often skipped. Your body does not know when you will feed it again, so it just stores EVERYTHING as fat. It stores it as fat so that if you skip meals your body feels it will have something to pull from.

These bad habits are not hard to break, and truly your body wants to work with you! So start eating less food, more often! If you are used to the second scenario, I have to warn you, you will most likely gain weight the first 1-2 weeks, because your body is still in "starvation/store mode."

After 1-2 weeks your body will start to trust you will continue to feed it and will really start working for you! Again, the only way to turn on your metabolism is by eating or working out.

As long as I brought up working out, let me tell you one other quick thing about eating and working out. Your body converts carbohydrates, fats and proteins into energy. However, it converts carbohydrates into energy the quickest and easiest, therefore it will burn through carbs quickest, then fats and proteins last. If you want to lose body fat, you need to do cardio on an empty stomach so your body is forced to pull from your body fat. If you have a carb in your body, it will pull from that for energy instead of your body-fat. Now the opposite is true about weight lifting. If you think about your body being like a car, a car can't run without gas, and your body can't run without carbs. When you are lifting, your body needs carbs for its gas, or energy. So again, cardio on an empty stomach, weight training after eating a carb.

The only way to burn through a carb is by moving, so eat these earlier in the day when you are up and active. Avoid those 3-4 hours before bed. I recommend avoiding carbs, fats, and fruits before bed. There are some exceptions. Someone trying to put on weight or size should include a carb with dinner. I also feel most young **children** still need carbs with dinner to keep them full through their long sleep hours.

CHAPTER 2
Meal Prepping

I am a single mom of two kids and cooking 4-6 meals a day every day just is out of the question for me. I love to cook in bulk! I typically make a huge batch of chicken, brown rice and green beans. I also always have fresh cut lettuce and fresh veggies. These are staples that I ALWAYS have on hand- a cooked carb, a cooked protein and a cooked veggie, along with at least one fresh veggie. Making meals becomes very easy when you already have everything cooked. A couple days you can have rice, chicken, and green beans. That night up can add rice and lettuce. Maybe the next day you make whole wheat noodles, and have a pasta salad with noodles, (already cooked chicken) and cut tomatoes. Noodles only take about 5-8 minutes to cook which is a lot easier then 30-45 minutes to cook chicken. With at least one carb, a protein and veggie always cooked, it makes making meals very easy, even if you want to mix it up during the week. You can also add different seasonings or dressings to make it taste different.

How to figure out how much to make:

If you're like me, you hate throwing food away!! I will use my family as an example. I eat 4oz of chicken 3-4 meals a day (but I will do the math at 3 meals a day)

- ✔ 4oz X 3meals a day= 12oz a day
- ✔ My kids eat 1-2 oz. a day 2 meals a day, and I have 2 kids
- ✔ 1oz X 2 meals a day X 2 kids= 4oz a day

- ✔ If I take that 12oz I eat and the 4oz my kids eat that's 16 oz. a day, times that by 5 days and its 80oz.

I buy my chicken at Costco. I like the frozen tenders. They come in a bag of 60oz. I put 1½ bags of frozen tenders in the Instant Pot. If you don't have an Instant Pot, I highly recommend you getting one, or a crock pot. I put the chicken in, add a lot of seasonings for flavor, add some water, put the lid on, and walk away. The Instant pot will cook it all in about 30-45 minutes. I will put it all in a Tupperware. I work from home so it is easy for me to get that out and make meals with it. However, if you don't work from home, I would suggest when your chicken is done, you measure it out, and using my example, put 4oz in 5 different containers. You can then add your carbs and veggies for lunches. There you have 5 packaged healthy lunches ready for the whole week, and all you have to do is grab a container in the morning and go. The remaining chicken can all go in a big Tupperware, and again, grab it out and measure it out for your next meal.

Now the same goes for your carbs. Using the example

of my kids and I again, I eat 3 carb meals a day in winter (when I'm less active) and 4 carb meals a day during the summer (when I'm much more active). I eat ½ c carbs with those carb meals. I eat oatmeal every morning for breakfast, as does my son, and it is my favorite meal of the day! That leaves me with 2 other carb meals a day. My kids will also have 4 carb meals a day, oatmeal being number 1, which leaves 3 other carb meals for them. My kids are like any other kids and don't want rice for every meal, so I will often make them a sandwich for one of the meals, or make noodles for one of the meals. My kids eat about ¼ cup of carbs per meal.

- ✔ ½ c carbs X 2 meals a day= 1 cup
- ✔ ¼ c carbs x 2 meals a day= ½ cup
- ✔ 1 cup for me + ½ c for them= 1 ½ cups
- ✔ 1 ½ cups times 5 days= 7 ½ cups of carbs

If I cook brown rice, 1 cup of dry rice will expand to about 3 cups cooked. If I need 7 ½ cups of rice, I measure out 2 ½ cups of dry rice. I put my rice in a rice cooker, add seasonings, add water, set the brown rice setting, and again walk away until it beeps and tells me it's done. Rice, couscous, and quinoa will expand like this. Spaghetti squash, butternut squash, sweet potatoes, red potatoes, etc. will not expand! So when cooking these things, I kind of eyeball the food and try to estimate what a cup of sweet potatoes would look like, and make the amount I will need. A medium sweet potato is about 1 cup.

Things I highly recommend to make your life easier:

- ✔ Instant Pot or Crockpot
- ✔ Rice Cooker
- ✔ Microwavable Vegetable Steamer

CHAPTER 3

Understanding Foods

When buying Proteins

Proteins should be low fat and low to no carbs. Lean meats are what you want to stick with! Use ground turkey instead of real hamburger, or turkey bacon instead of bacon. Try to avoid the yoke of the eggs, because they are full of cholesterol. The white part has no fat and is pure protein. If you love your yokes, try to do 3-5 whites to 1 yoke. When buying and using protein powders look for proteins with low carbs and low sugars (under 5 grams). Unless you are going to be using protein powders as a meal replacement, in which case you would want one with 20+ carbs. I like to eat my carbs so I don't do meal replacements. Although they can be great options for anyone working long hours, who don't have the ability to stop and eat every 2-3 hours.

When buying carbs

Make sure it's **a Whole Grain**

Look for the word "whole" before ingredient, whole wheat, whole rye, whole oats, and whole grain barley.

Other good whole grain choices- brown rice, buckwheat, couscous, oatmeal, quinoa, rolled oats, 100% whole wheat, 100% whole grain

Avoid foods with the following:

100% wheat, multi grain, contains whole grain, 7 grains, cracked wheat, made with whole grain, made with whole wheat, bran, unbleached, wheat flour

Please read not only the nutrition info, but also the ingredients. If you see any of these words from the avoid list in the ingredients pick a different product.

Your body will burn through and store a white, or unbleached carb the same as sugar, so try to avoid them!

When reading food labels look for the sugars (unless nature sugar like fruits), look for foods with 5g or less of sugar.

What's the purpose of it anyway???

CARBS (give your body energy, feed your brain, and help with memory)

Eat these earlier in the day, and limit these to your specific carb amount

Healthier carbs- oatmeal, sweet potatoes, black beans, couscous, quinoa, rice cakes, brown rice, spaghetti and acorn squash

Secondary carbs- whole wheat pastas, whole wheat breads, whole wheat crackers-(triscuits, wheat thins), low sugar cereal, red potatoes, protein bars

Your body will process the "healthier carbs" more efficiently then the "secondary carbs." If you are trying to lose weight, I highly recommend you stick primarily with the healthier carbs and use the secondary carbs sparingly (maybe 1 every 3-4 days). Once you are at your goal weight, and enjoying maintenance, you can enjoy more from the secondary list. Make sure they are still low in sugars and a whole healthy carb!

PROTEINS - helps build muscle

EAT THESE WITH EVERY MEAL. Your body can burn through proteins in your sleep. When hungry eat more proteins and veggies

Healthy proteins: fish, tuna, chicken, egg whites, protein powders, fresh deli meat (turkey), ground turkey, lean steak

When reading food labels, make sure your meats are low fat and low to no carbs.

DAIRY- builds and strengthens bones
(1-2 SERVINGS A DAY)

Healthy Dairy: fat free cottage cheese, yogurt or Greek yogurt, unsweetened almond milk, cheese (white, or unprocessed)

Be aware that regular milk, even fat free milk still has 16 grams of sugar per cup! Now I am not a milk drinker and never have been, but my son loves it, and I do buy him whole milk. Please remember while you are reading this, there are exceptions for many different people. And please remember a lot of this pertains to adults and how we should eat.

Also, with your yogurt, be sure and look at the sugar grams. Many yogurts are loaded with sugar, but they do have some that are better than others. I have found that Dannon Light and Fit taste good and have lower sugars then some.

VEGGIES and FRUITS- give your body needed vitamins and minerals

Veggies: tomatoes, carrots, Brussel sprouts, green beans, cucumbers, lettuce, spinach, yellow squash, zucchini, bell peppers, cauliflower, kale, celery, etc. (EAT AS MANY OF THESE AS YOU WANT)

Green veggies are better at nighttime.

Fruits: apples, oranges, bananas, mangoes, cantaloupe, watermelon, pineapple, melon, strawberries, raspberries, blueberries, etc. (AS ADULTS LIMIT TO 1-2 A DAY)

FAT (good fats help fit the bad fats)

Read food labels. Look for monounsaturated and polyunsaturated fats. These are the good ones.

Avoid saturated fats and Trans fats

Healthy Fats: All natural PB, avocados, almonds, cashews, avocado oil, coconut oil

Use fats sparingly, even the good ones. Avoid cooking with oil whenever you can, and try to use Pam sprays instead.

SUGARS (avoid them)

You want to avoid sugars unless from fruits as much as possible. Did you know there are over 50 different names for sugar?!?! So it's not as simple as reading a food label and looking for sugar any more. You need to de-code all their secretive names as well. As one of my clients stated, "What tricky little buggers!" And that's exactly what they are! I am going to be honest with you when I tell you; this whole sugar thing is still a challenge for me! Knowing all the different names to look for is overwhelming! But here is an easy key that will help you; almost ALL processed food has added sugar! Whereas whole foods will not! When you read a food label and you see more than 5g of sugar and it's not a fruit, you can pretty much guarantee its sugar you want to avoid! I am going to go over sugar a little more, and like I said it can be a little overwhelming. Here are 61 different names you will find sugar being called when reading a food label (ingredients)... Agave nectar, Barbados sugar, Barley malt, Barley malt syrup, Beet sugar, Brown sugar, Buttered syrup, Cane juice, Cane juice crystals, Cane sugar, Caramel, Carob syrup, Castor sugar, Coconut palm sugar, Coconut sugar, Confectioner's sugar, Corn sweetener, Corn syrup, Corn syrup solids, Date sugar, Dehydrated cane juice, Demerara sugar, Dextrin, Dextrose, Evaporated cane juice, Free-flowing brown sugars, Fructose, Fruit juice, Fruit juice concentrate, Glucose, Glucose solids, Golden sugar, Golden syrup, Grape sugar, HFCS (High-Fructose Corn Syrup), Honey, Icing sugar, Invert sugar, Malt syrup, Maltodextrin, Maltol, Maltose, Mannose, Maple syrup, Molasses, Muscovado, Palm sugar, Panocha, Powdered sugar, Raw sugar, Refiner's syrup, Rice syrup, Saccharose, Sorghum Syrup, Sucrose, Sugar (granulated),Sweet Sorghum, Syrup, Treacle, Turbinado sugar, Yellow sugar.

Overwhelmed yet?? Like I said it's overwhelming to me! But sticking with more natural whole foods and less processed foods will help a ton!

Added sugar is just what it says, added sugar to flavor a product. Did you know on average most adults eat 57 pounds of added sugars a year? Added sugars are usually a mixture of simple sugars such as glucose, fructose or sucrose. High-fructose added sugars are more harmful to your body then glucose. High-fructose sugars are processed in the liver, while the others are processed through all your cells. Sucrose is also known as table sugar. It occurs naturally in many fruits and plants, and is added to all sorts of processed foods. It consists of 50% glucose and 50% fructose. High-fructose corn syrup is produced from corn starch. It consists of varying amounts of fructose and glucose, but the most common type contains 55% fructose and 45% glucose.

There are no guidelines for a minimum amount of sugar intake, duh right... However, this is a limit to the max they recommend you get from added sugars each day. The American Heart Association recommends no more than 38 grams of added sugar a day for men and 25 grams of added sugar a day for women. Let me restate that, that does NOT say women eat at least 25 grams. It says eat as little added sugar as you can in a day, and especially do not go over those numbers.

Many Healthy foods have added sugar as well, like yogurts, milk, whole grain fruit bars, etc. So Please read your food labels and try to pick more foods without sugars, or low sugars.

CHAPTER 4

Reading a Food Label

Nutrition Facts

Serving Size 1 cup (228g)
Servings Per Container 2

(1) Start Here ➜

(2) Check Calories

Amount Per Serving

Calories 250   Calories from Fat 110

	% Daily Value*
Total Fat 12g	18%
Saturated Fat 3g	15%
Trans Fat 3g	
Cholesterol 30mg	10%
Sodium 470mg	20%
Total Carbohydrate 31g	10%
Dietary Fiber 0g	0%
Sugars 5g	
Protein 5g	
Vitamin A	4%
Vitamin C	2%
Calcium	20%
Iron	4%

(3) Limit these Nutrients

(4) Get Enough of these Nutrients

(6) Quick Guide to % DV

• 5% or less is Low

• 20% or more is High

* Percent Daily Values are based on a 2,000 calorie diet. Your Daily Values may be higher or lower depending on your calorie needs.

	Calories:	2,000	2,500
Total Fat	Less than	65g	80g
Sat Fat	Less than	20g	25g
Cholesterol	Less than	300mg	300mg
Sodium	Less than	2,400mg	2,400mg
Total Carbohydrate		300g	375g
Dietary Fiber		25g	30g

(5) **Footnote**

1. Check the serving size. Many times we look at a label and think, "Oh that isn't too bad." Unfortunately, a lot of times they break the servings size down so small you don't realize what your reading is for ¼ a candy bar and you ate the whole thing! The serving size is different on all things, so look at it, and then it will tell you how many servings are in the whole package. For the example above there are 2 servings in one package, so you would double every number you see if you had the whole thing.

2. Check the calories and see how many calories it has per serving and figure out how many servings you will be having

3. Look at the fat amount. Keep these numbers low, and make sure the fat is coming from monounsaturated or polyunsaturated fats and not trans-fat or saturated fats. Also look for the sugar amounts. You want to pick foods with 5g of sugar or less (unless fruits which are natural sugars)

4. Look for foods rich in nutrients

I like to add to this. After you have read the food label, make sure you also read the ingredients. I have already talked about things to look for.

CHAPTER 5

Portion Sizes

How much do you really need?

On average, adult women- ½ c carbs with 2-4 meals a day, 3-4oz meat (15-24 grams' protein) 4-6 meals a day

On average, adult men- 1 c carbs with 2-4 meals a day, 4-6oz meat (24-35 grams' protein) 4-6 meals a day

Sample Menu for an adult (you can also add a dairy just about anywhere here)

- ✔ Breakfast- carb, protein, fat
- ✔ Snack- protein, fruit, carb
- ✔ Lunch- protein, carb, veggie
- ✔ Snack- protein, veggie, fat (possible a carb)
- ✔ Dinner- protein, veggie
- ✔ Snack- protein (could add veggie)

As you can see in the above example, you want proteins with 4-6 meals a day, carbs fats and fruits earlier in the day. You can eat veggies or dairy any time of day, although yogurt can be high in sugars, so you may want to avoid them right before bed.

Here are some more examples of meal plans-

This is based off about 1500 calorie meal plan which most women fall into this range. This is geared for someone who wants to lose weight/fat and works out 30-45 minutes a day 3-5 days a week.

Pick one meal from each group every 2-3 hours.

Breakfast options

You could eat any food from any food group here

- ✔ ½ c oatmeal, cook then add 1 TBSP all natural PB, and 1 scoop protein, 1 fruit
- ✔ ½ c oatmeal cooked with stevia and cinnamon, 4 egg whites (scrambled, omelet, hard boiled), 1 fruit
- ✔ 1 Greek yogurt with ¼ c granola, 2 egg whites, 1 fruit
- ✔ Smoothie (1 Greek yogurt, ½ c oatmeal, 1TBSP PB, ½ c fruit, 1 scoop protein powder)
- ✔ ½ c red potatoes (in recipes), 4 egg whites, fruit
- ✔ 4 egg whites, 1 whole wheat tortilla, fruit

AM snack: (You could eat fruit here instead of with breakfast, but 1 fruit a day.)

You can eat food from any food group here

- ✔ 1 Greek yogurt, 2 rice cakes, 15 almonds

- 1 c fat free cottage cheese, 2 rice cakes, 15 almonds
- Protein bar, 1/8 c nuts
- ¼c carb (rice, sweet potatoes, black beans, couscous), 4oz meat, 1/8 avocado
- 5 crackers, 15 nuts, protein shake

Lunch:

Carb, protein, veggie (You could also add a fat if haven't already gotten 2 in)

- ½ c squash, 4oz meat, or fish, 1 c veggies
- ½ c brown rice, 4oz meat or fish, 1 c veggie
- ½ c beans, 3oz meat or fish, 1 c veggies
- ½ c couscous, 4oz meat or fish, 1 c veggies
- ½ c carb, 4oz meat (or protein scoop), 1 c veggies
- 2 slice bread, 4oz meat, 1 cup veggies
- ½ c pasta, 4oz meat, 1 cup veggies

Snack:

Protein and veggie (You could do a carb here if you haven't already gotten 2-3 carbs in, could also add a fat if haven't already gotten 2 in)

- 3oz meat, 1 c veggies
- Protein shake, 1 c veggies
- 4 egg whites, 1 c veggies

Dinner: 3-4 hours before bed

- ✔ Any protein and veggies
- ✔ 4oz meat or fish, 1 c veggie
- ✔ 5 egg whites, 1 c veggies

Pm Snack: (If hungry before bed)

- ✔ Any protein
- ✔ Protein shake
- ✔ 2-3oz meat
- ✔ 2-3 egg whites

If you would like a specific meal plan to follow based on your goals, please feel free to message me, Amara@ TeamCrazyFit.com

Chapter 6

Fad Diets

I personally don't recommend fad diets, although they are a GREAT way to lose weight fast. It is not something you can stick with long term, nor are they healthy for you to stick with long term. I often see people go on a fad diet, lose weight, then fall of the diet because they are too hard to maintain and gain everything they lost plus 10 extra pounds. Cutting carbs completely out of your diet is extremely damaging to your body in the long term. Your body will forget how to process them and it slows your metabolism way down if kept too low for too long. So please don't cut carbs out of your diet, just switch to the healthier ones and eat them earlier in the day. I also understand that to quickly lose weight cutting carbs does help, so I recommend two things.

1. You cut carbs after a cheat day (if you ate more junk then you should have). Cutting your carbs, the next day in half helps even it out. But then you get back to your regular plan by the second or third day

2. Carb cycling: This means high or normal amount of carbs one day followed by 1-2 days of low carbs. It is extremely effective in helping you lose weight without damaging your metabolism.

This is also based on a 1500 calorie diet

First 2 weeks' low carb. If energy levels get too low during these 2 weeks, add ¼ c carb with morning snack on low day.

Carbs: Pick from healthy carb list
No secondary carbs, or limit it to 1-2 a week
LOW carb

Breakfast:

- ✔ ¼ c healthy carbs, 1sc protein, 1 fruit, 1 ½ tbsp PB
- ✔ ¼ c healthy carbs, 7 egg whites, 1 fruit, ¼ avocado
- ✔ 1 English muffin, 7 egg whites, 1 fruit, ¼ avocado

Snack:

- ✔ 5oz meat, 30 almonds, yogurt (optional)
- ✔ 1 ½ protein shake with 8oz unsweetened almond milk, 30 almonds

Lunch:

- ¼ c healthy carbs, 4oz meat, 1 c veggies
- ½ tortilla, 4oz meat, 1 c veggies
- 2 rice cakes, 4oz meat, 1 c veggies

Snack:

- 5oz meat, 1 c veggies, ¼ avocado
- 5oz meat, 1 cup veggies, 30 almonds/nuts
- 1 ½ scoop protein, 1 c veggies

Dinner:

- 5oz meat, 1 c veggies
- 1 ½ scoop protein, 1 c veggies

Snack:

- 4oz meat
- 1 scoop protein shake

HIGH or REG DAY

Breakfast:

- ½ c carbs, 1 scoop protein, 1 fruit, 1 ½ tbsp. PB
- ½ c carbs, 6 egg whites, 1 fruit, ¼ avocado
- 1 whole English muffin, 6 egg whites, 1 fruit, ¼ avocado

Snack:

- ½ c carbs, 3oz meat, yogurt (optional)
- 3 rice cakes, 1 protein shake with 8oz unsweetened almond milk, 30 almonds
- 1 tortilla, 3oz meat, ¼ avocado

Lunch:

- ½ c carbs, 3oz meat, 1 c veggies
- 1 tortilla, 3oz meat, 1 c veggies
- 4 rice cakes, 4oz meat, 1 c veggies

Snack: -

- 4oz meat, 1 c veggies, ¼ avocado
- 4oz meat, 1 cup veggies, 30 almonds/nuts
- 1 scoop protein, 1 c veggies

Dinner:

- 4oz meat, 1 c veggies
- 1 scoop protein, 1 c veggies

Snack:

- 3oz meat
- 1 scoop protein shake

Chapter 7
Food Journal

Keep a food journal- This is such a powerful tool! Write down everything you eat; the amount and the time. I like to have emotional eaters write down how you are feeling when you eat as well. Hungry? Angry? Stressed? Bored? (And let's be honest, we are all emotional eaters at times). Most people do not realize how much they eat each day, and how much bad stuff you eat each day, myself included. During the holidays I start snacking on treats a little here and there, but before I know it I've gained 5-8 pounds in just a few weeks. I do this every year, and by the beginning of January, I realize my snack and junk food eating has gotten a little out of control.

I start a food journal to really help me be accountable for what I eat. How often do you eat a meal and then walk into the pantry and grab a handful of nuts, or trail mix with M&M's, or a handful of chips? Or walk past a co-worker's desk and grab a handful of M&Ms or Hershey kisses? Even with something healthy, the handfuls add up quickly. You may be eating an extra 200-1000 calories a day that you are not even thinking about! Like I said I AM just as guilty at this! I eat breakfast (oatmeal, protein and Peanut Butter) and often find myself raiding the pantry when I get done, even though I am not hungry. It's just a habit (especially after the holidays of eating so much)! A helpful tool for getting back on track is to keep a food journal!

Have a notebook in the kitchen or keep a log in your notes on your phone, whatever works for you. Every time you eat, write down what you eat, including how much and what time. If you want to go grab a handful of nuts, you need to write that down. If you go back for another handful, write that down as well! When doing this often, I think to myself, "I don't really want to have to write down I ate a handful of nuts, again and again and again." I can look at my food journal and realize I just ate 20 minutes ago so I'm probably not really hungry and try to decide why I'm going to snack. Am I bored? Anxious, mad or sad?

I am getting a little sidetracked here, but I do want you to realize how important keeping a food journal is. Again write down everything you eat, including the amount and the time. You can take it a step further and find a partner for this and the two of you can exchange your food journals every week. Knowing someone is going to look over what you eat will also help you make better eating choices. You don't really want someone to know you ate 6 cookies in one sitting. Post your food journal on social media for accountability or just keep track for yourself, whatever works best for you. Just be honest on it, write down everything. I promise it will bring such an awareness of what you are eating to yourself that you did not know or realize before.

CHAPTER 8

Substitutes

Use Pam as much as possible and avoid oils when cooking. The fats add up quickly even with healthy oils. If you do not like nuts, or avocado then oils are a good option for your daily healthy fat. However, if you are already getting your fat from other forms, try to avoid them when cooking.

Use seasonings for flavor instead of dressings and sauces. Buy 1-2 new seasonings every week to try. I love salad supreme, lemon pepper, taco seasoning, and bbq seasonings.

Buy sugar free dressings.

Replace butter with water when cooking (or use half water half butter and find a healthier alternative to butter, like Smart balance butter, or I can't believe it's not butter, butter). I often use plain yogurt instead of butter as well, or applesauce.

Use Stevia for sweetening, instead of Sugar or Splenda.

CHAPTER 9

Eating Out

Eating out is convenient and fun, but make it something special, not an everyday occurrence.

There really is NO way to meet your health goals eating out every day. We have talked about meal prepping, and once you get in the habit of doing this, it is much easier and cheaper than eating out every day. Also instead of taking an hour to go to lunch, you can eat in 10 minutes, take a shorter lunch, and use the remanding time to get a 30-40-minute workout in. If you must eat out, here are my recommendations:

Order salads whenever you can. Get grilled chicken instead of fried. Ask for your dressing on the side (ask for fat free dressing options, many restaurants have them or at least reduced fat options). If salad comes with bacon, chips, croutons, or any other fattening unhealthy ingredients, and you can't live without it, ask for it on the side as well. You can put some on but maybe not all of it.

Order all food without butter. At breakfast, your pancakes come with a glob of butter or your toast comes with butter already melted on it. Veggies are cooked in lots of butter. Ask for these options without butter. A simple "Can I get that without butter please?" is all it takes.

Meat and veggies are always good options. Again, ask that it be cooked without butter, and again, grilled not fried.

Be aware that most restaurants are using white or unbleached noodles, bread, rice, etc.unless it is a healthy restaurant, and they specify that it is brown rice or whole grain bread.

CHAPTER 10
Night Time Binging

I hear over and over from clients, and myself included, that nighttime is the hardest time to stick with the meal plan. Your body and mind have done one of two things today. You have been so busy you haven't had a chance to think about cheating, but now your home, things have slowed down and you start thinking a bowl of popcorn sounds good, or a bowl of ice cream, or whatever that cheat food is for you. The second thing is you have been craving a treat all day long and resisting. Someone brought in donuts and you turned it down. Someone else invited you to pizza for lunch and you turned it down. You walked past the jar of M&M's all day long and passed up on them. Now you are home and you're tired and you just have no will-power left and you cave! I don't have a magic pill that makes your cravings go away, or makes your sweet tooth go away, although I do swear by some fat burner/appetite suppressant pills to help with cravings that I will mention in a minute). Here are some things that help me with cravings:

1. Drink 8-10oz of water quickly it will fill your stomach up and make you feel full. We often as humans' mistake thirst for hunger. Make sure you are drinking enough water throughout the day!

2. Brush your teeth after dinner, I'm lazy, or efficient, however you want to look at it, however I don't want to do the same thing twice. So after dinner I floss and brush and just know I'm done eating for the night. Sometimes I come back down and really want something else but then think I really don't want to brush my teeth again, so I pass.

3. Try some natural fat burner/appetite suppressants. I have a few I love, and rotate through every 2-3 months. I love Team Crazy Fit Influence (all natural), Muscle Pharm Shredded Sport, and Cellucor Super HD. I always take a few months off these pills, typically November-January/February and start back up February/March with Influence for 2 months, then Shredded Sport 2 months, then Super HD for 2 months. These truly help me not crave junk food, and I really do have the biggest sweet tooth!

CHAPTER 11

It's Up to You

Make eating healthy a choice for your whole family. It is up to YOU as parents to feed your children healthy food and educate them of what healthy food is. I hear all the time parents who say my kids will only eat Macaroni and Cheese or Top Ramon. Trust me when I say your kids will NOT starve if they choose to miss a meal or two. Most parents decide they are going to start eating healthier, but the kids don't want it, so these sweet, kind, loving parents don't want their kids to starve, so they break down and make the mac n cheese, but don't do it! Your kids may refuse to eat healthy food, but eventually they will get hungry and have it. So don't give in, make the choice to be healthier, for you and your family! It's your responsibility to stock your fridge and pantry with healthy food your kids can eat, at just about any time they want. My four and six-year-old will often open the fridge on their own and grab an apple, orange, some carrots, or a yogurt. There isn't anything in my fridge or pantry that my kids can't, for the most part, have at any time. I know as your kids get older, it's out of your control what they eat a lot of the time. That is another reason to really teach them what healthy food is and how to enjoy it, and have it as their only options when they are home.

CHAPTER 12

Simple Meal Plans

Weekly Meal Plan

With the information above about meal prepping and measuring out how much food to make, here's an example of a weekly meal plan for you and family if you cooked mixed veggies, green beans, rice, chicken and egg whites at start of week and made ground turkey, peas and sweet potatoes towards the end or middle of the week (or you could make this all at the start of the week).

I know this doesn't give a WHOLE lot of variety, but it is easy! If you are someone who wants to cook dinner every night, by all means do so, I have included many recipes and you could pick a different one every night. This just shows you how easy it can be to truly cook 1-2 times a week for the whole week.

Day 1

- ✔ Breakfast: Oatmeal with Peanut Butter (I personally make each bowl separately. I make my son's with whole milk, my daughter's with almond milk and mine with water.) I put a huge heaping tablespoon of all natural Peanut Butter in both my kid's oatmeal and then cook in microwave for 45-80 seconds. I add a scoop of Muscle Pharm protein to mine, and about ½0 scoop to my kids
- ✔ Snack: yogurt and apple, 2 rice cakes with Peanut Butter
- ✔ Lunch: chicken rice and veggies that were already pre-cooked earlier for meal prepping
- ✔ Snack: adults- chicken and rice, possibly add rice (already pre-cooked)
- ✔ Kids: apple with PB
- ✔ Dinner: adults- chicken, lettuce and sugar free dressing
- ✔ Kids: chicken, lettuce and sugar free dressing, BBQ chicken pita pizzas (with chicken that was already made)

Day 2

- ✔ Breakfast: Kodiak cake pancake mix (make enough for 2 days' worth) top with Peanut Butter and sugar free syrup or Kodiak cakes all natural syrup
- ✔ Snack: Peanut Butter balls, apple
- ✔ Lunch: Pita bread Peanut Butter and jelly

sandwiches and carrot sticks

- ✔ Snacks: adults-protein shake, salad with sugar free dressing
- ✔ Kids: apple and Peanut Butter and rice cakes
- ✔ Dinner: adults- chicken and green beans (cooked in advance) use teriyaki sauce as dressing or a sugar free dressing, could melt cheese on chicken as well
- ✔ Kids: chicken and green beans, noodles (cooked fresh 2-3 nights worth), add cheese and teriyaki sauce

Day 3

- ✔ Breakfast: pancakes again
- ✔ Snack: yogurt add raspberries and granola to yogurt
- ✔ Lunch: noodles from last night, turkey pepperonis, chicken, cut carrots, green beans, olives, parmesan cheese and fat free Italian dressing, and salad supreme seasoning
- ✔ Snack: chicken lettuce salad (optional carb), sugar free dressing
- ✔ Kids: orange, apples, carrot sticks and wheat thins
- ✔ Dinner: adults-egg whites and mixed veggies
- ✔ Kids: egg whites, rice, mixed veggies

Day 4

- ✔ Breakfast: whole wheat toast with Peanut Butter on top and egg whites with cheese and avocado

- ✔ Snack: Peanut Butter balls, banana
- ✔ Lunch: chicken and rice and green beans
- ✔ Snack: adults-egg whites and veggies (add rice possibly)
- ✔ Kids: above add strawberries
- ✔ Dinner: adults- chicken, lettuce, turkey pepperonis, parmesan cheese, cut dill pickles, fat free Italian dressing
- ✔ Kids: above salad, add rice

Day 5

- ✔ Breakfast: oatmeal again
- ✔ Snack: yogurt, apple, Peanut Butter
- ✔ Lunch: egg whites, sweet potatoes, cheese and peas
- ✔ Snack: adults-chicken, lettuce and low fat honey mustard
- ✔ Kids: apples and bananas, snap peas, mini rice cakes
- ✔ Dinner: 99% fat free ground turkey (cooked with taco seasoning), cheese, lettuce and salsa
- ✔ Kids: ground turkey, sweet potatoes cheese and peas

Day 6

- ✔ Breakfast: Kodiak cakes with Peanut Butter
- ✔ Snack: Peanut Butter balls apple
- ✔ Lunch: sweet potatoes and ground turkey, cheese, peas
- ✔ Snack: protein shake, carrot sticks (add carb possibly)

- Kids: carrot sticks, apples, chicken sandwiches on pita bread with cheese (warmed in microwave)
- Dinner: adults- eggs and green beans
- Kids: egg burrito with whole-wheat tortilla, cheese, green beans

Day 7

- Breakfast: oatmeal
- Snack: yogurt, nuts, apples
- Lunch: noodles, ground turkey, tomato sauce with garlic pepper and tomatoes
- Snack: adults-egg whites and peas
- Kids: apples and cheese quesadillas
- Dinner: adults-ground turkey, cheese lettuce and salsa
- Kids: pita pizza- with leftover tomato sauce and garlic pepper, turkey pepperonis and cheese, side salad.

CHAPTER 13

My Food Staples

My staple foods that we always have in stock

Fridge:

- Unsweetened vanilla almond milk (This is a great alternative to milk, also great with protein shakes)
- Eggs
- Liquid egg whites
- Dannon fit and light Greek yogurt
- Fresh fruit (we try to have at least two different kinds)
- Fresh veggies (at least 2 different kinds)
- Fresh lettuce (secret-buy the kind you cut yourself, and then cut enough for 2-3 days at a time, wash it and put it in a large zip lock bag. Get a new bag every time you cut and wash it. This will help it stay fresh longer, it only stays crisp for 2-3 days after its been cleaned and cut).

- Low fat mozzarella cheese
- Deli turkey
- Turkey pepperonis
- Skinny girl salad dressings- poppy seed, and balsamic vinaigrette
- Fat Free Italian dressing
- Teriyaki sauce (we love this although it is high in sugar so use it sparingly)
- Dill pickles
- Cooked chicken
- Cooked veggies
- Cooked carb

Freezer

- Frozen chicken
- Frozen 99% fat free ground turkey
- Frozen veggies
- Frozen fruit
- Bananas on a stick wrapped in tinfoil frozen (make super tasty popsicles)

Pantry

- Quaker rice cakes (large size- Caramel, chocolate, and tomatoes basil, plain)
- Quaker rice cakes (minis cheese, lime and ranch) (Be aware that the caramel minis are loaded with sugar!)
- Wheat thins/triscuits (some sort of whole wheat crackers)
- One-two low sugar cereals like cheerios, Life or Chex

- ✔ Almonds, and cashews
- ✔ Smart Balance All Natural Peanut Butter
- ✔ Protein powders (1 at a min, but I like 2-3 different flavors at all times). I love Muscle Pharm, but there are lots of great protein powders.
- ✔ Protein bars- I love Quest bars and Muscle Pharm Combat bars
- ✔ Kodiak cakes pancake batter (avoid the flavored ones they have a lot more sugar and really don't taste that much better. Stick with the original buttermilk mix)
- ✔ Sugar free syrup (when buying this, please read the label and make sure it does not have aspartame in it either! There are so many studies on the harmful effects of aspartame).
- ✔ Bars for my kids when out on the go or in a hurry (Cliff Zbars, Nature Valley bars, all natural fig or fruit bars, *(now like I mentioned before even healthy bars are loaded with sugar, so don't use these as a snack every day but work great if you are going to be in the car for a while or going out for the day.)*
- ✔ Papa Pita Greek pita flat bread 100% whole wheat (we use this instead of bread)
- ✔ Dried fruit, typically craisins (Dried fruit is loaded with extra sugar, so don't eat a lot of it, but it's great to put into trail mixes.

CHAPTER 14
The Sweet Tooth

Here are a few not so healthy staples, but a healthier alternative to the real thing.

- ✔ Popcorn kernels that we pop and flavor ourselves. I love to buy butter-flavored spray-zero calories and spray our popcorn with that and sprinkle sea-salt
- ✔ Dark chocolate chips make sure they have a cacao content of 70% or higher to be able to get some nutrients out of this tasty treat. I buy Pascha organic dark chocolate 85% cacao.

Now to be completely honest, I have the biggest sweet tooth, and I often wish I could eat whatever I wanted and still look the way I wanted to look. I love sweet baked goods, and I also really enjoy making them. I can't stand the thought of throwing them out, but also know it's probably not best to eat the whole batch of cookies in one setting. So here's the secret. I make a batch and have one or two or maybe even three, ha-ha, but then I take the rest, put them in a zip lock freezer bag, and freeze them.

I truly eat very healthy 10-11 months out of the year, but even when I am eating healthy, I like to have a cheat once a week. Having a bag of frozen cookies, or cupcakes, or even my kids store bought birthday cakes in the freezer allows me to do two things:

1. Plan ahead: I have to think out beforehand that I'm going to cheat, and what I want to cheat on. Do you know that planning out your cheat allows you to be able to enjoy it a lot more? You don't feel guilty that you gave in and couldn't fight the urge any more. You full on woke up that morning and said today is my cheat day and I'm going to have a chocolate chip cookie later today. The reason you have to plan ahead is because it's frozen, so you have to give it a few hours to thaw out so you can eat it. I can grab 1 cookie out, put it in a small Ziploc bag on the counter and let it air thaw. When it's thawed, it tastes just as good as when you bought it, or made it!

2. Having frozen treats in your freezer keeps you from having to buy a whole cake because you want one piece, or make a whole batch of cookies because you want one cookie. I eat so many more cookies when I am making them than when I have to pull one out of the freezer. Many people say they would eat them all the time if they knew they were there. If they were in my pantry I would as well, but that's your

binge eating, that completely out of control, typically emotional eating. Pulling them out of freezer and thawing them to eat a planned treat, is the complete opposite of that, and really does make you feel more in control of your eating.

CHAPTER 15

Positive I AM Affirmation

Positive I AM affirmation around eating and body image. Of course you can use positive affirmations in all areas of life, but again the purpose of this book is for better health so I am going to give you examples of positive affirmations in this area.

I AM healthy
I AM in perfect health
I AM at my goal weight of _____
I AM always in control of what I eat
I AM able to portion control always
I love my body
I AM perfect just the way I am
I AM getting better and better every day in every way

These are just a few of my favorites, but feel free to write your own as well. Make sure your positive affirmations are written as if you already have what you want, and also make sure you are writing what you DO want, and not what you DON'T want. Example I am at my perfect weight; vs I don't want to be overweight. Read these positive affirmations every day. I also recommend you writing a statement about what your ideal health and fitness would look like, how you will feel if you were at your ideal body weight, how you would look, what you would do and what you would eat. Write these feelings down as fast as they come to you and then rewrite them in sentences and in a positive form, like you are already there, then again read this out loud 2 times a day, and truly feel the feeling of being at your ideal weight, and perfect health. Find Pictures of bodies you want your body to look like, and glue them to paper, along with some of your I AM affirmations and look at that as often as you can. Tape your goal weight on your scale so when you step on it all you see is your goal weight.

CHAPTER 16

10 Minute Meal Recipes

Sweet potatoes- cook at 425 in oven- poke holes in sweet potatoes with fork, wrapped in tinfoil, place on cooking sheet. For easy clean up, I always wrap my cookie sheet in tin foil before cooking anything on it. Depending how many sweet potatoes you have, cook for 30-45 minutes, stick a fork in them to see if they are done, if they are soft they are done.

- ✔ another way to cook sweet potatoes, dice the sweet potatoes and again wrapped in tinfoil and cook on 425 for 20-40 minutes. I will sometimes sprinkle cinnamon on these after I cut them, before you cook them, which is super good and makes them a little more like a treat.

Rice- I already mentioned how to measure out how much rice you want to cook, but here's the final touches. Add seasonings to your rice, and don't be afraid to REALLY season it! Some of my favorites-lemon pepper, salad supreme, and taco seasoning, then you want to double the amount of water in cups of dry rice, so if you put 4 cups dry rice you will put about 8 cups of water

10 min Meal ideas-

I know I have already said this, but again I already cooked the meat, carb and veggie in advance. Then I can easily throw these meals together.

<u>Sweet potatoes</u>

- ✔ sweet potatoes, ground turkey (cooked with taco seasoning), low fat mozzarella cheese, cooked peas (or you could use tomatoes or another veggie of your choice) microwave for 30-60 seconds
- ✔ Sweet potatoes, chicken, green beans, add teriyaki sauce microwave for 30-60 seconds
- ✔ -Sweet potatoes, egg whites, peas microwave for 30-60 seconds

<u>Noodles-</u> (noodles only take about 8-10 minutes to cook so when I cook these I make enough for 2-3 meals)

- ✔ noodles, chicken, tomatoes, turkey pepperonis, salad supreme seasonings, fat free Italian dressing
- ✔ noodles, chicken, low fat mozzarella cheese, teriyaki sauce, green beans (or other veggie- I actually love this combo with lettuce as my veggie), microwave 30-60seconds

- Noodles, chicken, low fat mozzarella cheese, veggie, microwave 30-60 seconds
- chicken bouillon soup, I put a couple cubes of chicken bouillon in warm water and microwave for 2-3 minutes until hot and cube has dissolved, in a bowl put noodles, chicken, peas or carrots, add the chicken bouillon broth
- noodles, 99% fat free turkey burger, plain tomato sauce (I add garlic pepper to this), you could also add the low fat mozzarella cheese, tomatoes or peas go great with this, microwave

Rice-

- Rice, chicken, veggie teriyaki sauce, microwave 30-60 secs
- rice, chicken, lettuce, fat free dressing
- rice, eggs, veggie
- rice, ground turkey and veggie

Papa Pita Greek pita flat bread 100% whole wheat (we don't do much bread, but use theses a lot)

- Pita pizza- pita bread, spread bbq sauce, cooked chicken, low fat mozzarella cheese, microwave 45-60 seconds (until cheese melts), I typically add tomatoes on this or a salad on the side for veggie
- Pita pizza- tomato sauce (again add garlic pepper for flavoring), turkey pepperonis,

cheese (or any other toppings you enjoy), microwave 45-60 seconds
- ✔ Pita sandwiches- chicken and cheese and veggies, microwave the sandwich with chicken and cheese then add veggies to sandwich- lettuce, tomatoes, etc.

CHAPTER 17
Breakfasts

Kodiak cake pancakes- (I buy this at *Costco*, but you can also get on *Amazon*, and many different places). My secret: add a little vanilla extract and cinnamon, add water or decrease water depending what texture you want (directions on the back of the box).

Kodiak cake fruit pancakes-

✔ Make them like above and add raspberries, blueberries, or blackberries (could be fresh or frozen).

Kodiak cake pumpkin pancakes-

✔ Make like above but add canned pumpkin, could use pumpkin spice instead of cinnamon

Kodiak apple muffins-

✔ 3 cups Kodiak mix, 2 c almond milk, 2 eggs, cinnamon (mix)

✓ 3 apples peeled and chopped. Mix-1 single serving vanilla Dannon Fit and Light Greek yogurt, a splash of vanilla, then add apples, mix, then add to Kodiak mix, cook at 250 for 12-14 minutes (cook in cupcake tins with pam, do not use muffin liners they will stick to them)

Oatmeal- I like the Old Fashion Oats (NOT the instant or 1-minute kind)

I make mine with ½ cup dry oats, ½ cup water (you could use almond milk) and about ½ teaspoon of all natural *Smart Balance* Peanut Butter, microwave for 120 seconds, stir add another ¼c water to consistency, then add one scoop of *Muscle Pharm Combat Protein* my favorite flavors in oatmeal, chocolate or cookies and cream. DO NOT add the protein until after it is cooked, it will become a weird texture if you do.

Oatmeal for my children I primarily flavor with the Peanut Butter, so they get 1 heaping tablespoon of Peanut Butter, cook 45-120 seconds add more milk to texture (as mentioned before I use milk in my kid's oatmeal, because it gives it more flavor).

You can also add fruit to your oatmeal for flavor as well.

Papa Pita Greek flatbread fresh toast- 2 egg whites, 2 whole eggs, 1 tsp vanilla, a couple of shakes of cinnamon (mix): rip the bread into strips, soak in batter, cook on frying pan with Pam on medium

<u>Yogurt parfait</u>- *Dannon Light and Fit Greek* yogurt, frozen fruit (or fresh fruit), ¼-½ c dry oats (could use granola as well but again granola has sugar in it), ½-1 scoop chocolate protein (mix in the protein before adding any other ingredients).

-<u>Cottage cheese and yogurt</u>- ½ cup fat free cottage cheese, ½ c *Dannon Light and Fit Greek* yogurt, ½ scoop chocolate protein, mix then add ½ c frozen fruit

<u>Egg quiche</u>-

- ✔ 1 carton of liquid egg whites
- ✔ 6 pieces of turkey cut small
- ✔ 2 Bell peppers cut small, 1 cup spinach, ½ c low fat mozzarella cheese (any other veggies that sound good)
- ✔ Mix everything-pour into cupcake tins make at 350 for 25 minutes

<u>Thin omelet</u>-

- ✔ To make these thin and easy to snack on- I cook them on the griddle
- ✔ Spray griddle with pam- pour liquid egg white to cover the whole griddle
- ✔ Mix- turkey, spinach, tomatoes, shredded cheese (whatever else you want on it) pour mix on one side of the eggs. Once egg is cooked, take side without toppings and flip over side that has toppings, cut into squares

<u>Crepes</u>-

- ✔ Crepes- 1 c liquid egg whites

- ✔ ¼ c water
- ✔ 3 TBSP almond flour
- ✔ ½ scoop vanilla protein powder
- ✔ 2TBSP stevia
- ✔ (Mix all together- cook on frying pan with pam on low/med heat, pour mixture thin)
- ✔ Mixture- 1 single serving *Dannon Fit and Light* strawberry cheesecake Greek yogurt, 2 tbsp. low fat cream cheese (mix together) add fruit of your choice, roll up in crepe

Breakfast Potatoes-

Cube red potatoes, spray tin foil with Pam season with garlic pepper, wrap up and bake in the oven at 375 for 45-60 minutes.

Or

Cube red potatoes and cook them in microwave veggie steamer with water and garlic pepper

To make either recipe crunchier- after they are cooked put them on frying pan with pam on low/med heat, it will crisp the outside.

Egg-bake

Take a cake dish, pour egg whites ½ full cake pan, and 1 can chicken, season (any seasonings you like) stir, bake at 350 stirring occasionally, until the eggs are cooked and not liquid any more

CHAPTER **18**

Lunch

Egg/chicken scramble

Spray pan with pam, pour in eggs cook them until they are scrambled, then add chicken cook until chicken is browned (add seasonings to the liquid eggs, and again once you add chicken)

Quesadillas- melt cheese in microwave on whole wheat tortillas, the secret, turn your stove on medium/low and lightly toast each side (remember to spray pan with Pam). I add turkey to this often, and sometimes pepperonis, also once cooked and off the pan, I put lettuce in it (my son calls it the crunchy goodness.)

Tomato basil turkey rice cake- buy the tomato basil rice cakes, put a few slices of turkey and a slice of low fat mozzarella cheese on top of the turkey microwave for 20-30 seconds

Mango enchiladas-

- Cake dish- spray with pam lay down 2-3 whole wheat tortillas on bottom
- Middle- use chicken you have already cooked and cut into small pieces (or you can use 2 cans of canned chicken-drained) 12oz of chicken, ¼c low fat cream cheese, ½-1c frozen or fresh mangos (mix all together), layer on tortillas
- Enchilada packet- use ½ packet, ¼ c tomato sauce, ¼ c water (mix) use ¾ mixture on chicken
- Layer ¼-½c shredded mozzarella cheese
- Top with 2-3 more tortillas, pour remaining enchilada sauce, cover with tinfoil cook 325 for 30-45 minutes, uncover and cook until everything is melted.

Chicken Pea soup-

- 1 can cream of chicken 99% fat free
- 1 can unsweetened vanilla almond milk
- 1 cup frozen peas
- 1 can chicken (or 6oz chicken shredded)
- ½ c shredded mozzarella cheese
- Cook on pot med/high until warm add salt and seasoned pepper to taste

Teriyaki chicken noodles-

- 6oz chicken
- 1 cup snap peas, 1 cup cut carrots (cook on med/high on frying pan) with water and 2-4

tbsp. teriyaki sauce, once cooked add the chicken, mix together
- ✔ Costco's rice ramen noodles- 2 stacks of noodles cook in water- then toast on frying pan on low/med heat
- ✔ Add all together (add a little more teriyaki for flavoring if needed)

Pita Pizza- listed above as well

- ✔ 1 pita bread, 1-2 tbsp. BBQ sauce, spread, add 2-4oz chicken, and 1 tomato, top with mozzarella cheese microwave 1min or until cheese is melted
- ✔ Could also do this with tomato sauce (season with garlic pepper) top with turkey pepperonis, tomatoes, black olives and cheese

Healthy top ramen-

- ✔ Costco Ramon rice noodles (2 stacks), 2 cups water, 4 chicken bouillon cubes
- ✔ Cook until noodles are soft, add cooked shredded chicken, and cooked peas and carrots

Chicken burritos-

- ✔ 1 whole wheat tortilla, topped with 2-4oz chicken, black beans, cheese, fold and microwave for 45 seconds, then put on frying pan low/med heat to toast both sides.
- ✔ Black beans- soak overnight in taco seasoning and then cook in crock pot until soft.
- ✔ could also make this without beans

Cream of chicken spinach chicken-

- ✔ Bake chicken in cake pan with a can of cream of chicken soup, 1 can chicken broth
- ✔ Cook spinach on frying pan with water and salt and seasoned pepper
- ✔ Once chicken is cooked top chicken with spinach and some of the cream of chicken/ chicken broth mixture from chicken
- ✔ Toast a wheat bagel and put the chicken, spinach on top and melt some mozzarella cheese over it

Lasagna-

- ✔ 1 package 99% fat free ground turkey (cook on stove with taco seasoning) once cooked add a ½ can tomato sauce
- ✔ Mix- 2 cups fat free cottage cheese, 2 cups shredded low fat mozzarella cheese, 2 egg whites, 2 tbsp. Parmesan cheese
- ✔ In cake pan-pour ¼ c tomato sauce, lay down a layer of whole wheat lasagna noodles, then meat mixture, then cheese mixture, layer of noodles, repeat, layer of noodles, top with remaining ¼ can tomato sauce
- ✔ Bake at 350 for 45 minutes with tinfoil on, then 10 more minutes with tinfoil off

Turkey wraps-

Slice of turkey, top with a scoop of fat free cottage cheese, sliced tomato and dill pickle, wrap the turkey around it. Could add lettuce and make it a lettuce wrap

Chicken salad-

- ✔ 1 can canned chicken rinsed
- ✔ ½ c fat free cottage cheese, 1/8c low fat cream cheese, 2 cucumbers (peeled and cubed), 4-5 cut dill pickles, 5-10 cut red grapes (mix)
- ✔ Put on whole wheat bagel or whole wheat pita bread

Rice Cake Nachos-

- ✔ Small cheese or ranch rice cakes
- ✔ Top with refried black beans (or regular black beans)
- ✔ Shredded chicken, tomato, cheese (microwave) add black olives and salsa

Alfredo spaghetti squash-

- ✔ 1 whole spaghetti squash microwave for a few minutes until soft enough to cut
- ✔ Cut in half longwise, scoops all seeds out, flavor with sea salt and seasoned pepper cover with tinfoil- cook in oven at 425 for 15-30 minutes (until soft)
- ✔ Top with grilled chicken and Alfredo sauce.

Cauliflower rice bowl-

- ✔ Cook chicken in Instant Pot with salad supreme
- ✔ 1 bag cauliflower rice cooked
- ✔ 10-20 cherry tomatoes
- ✔ 20 snap peas

- ✔ 1 tsp fat free Italian dressing

Teriyaki noodle bowl-

- ✔ Whole wheat thin noodles cooked (1 cup)
- ✔ 10-20 cherry tomatoes
- ✔ 20 snap peas
- ✔ 1tbsp feta cheese
- ✔ 1tbsp teriyaki sauce
- ✔ 4oz chicken cooked with salad supreme seasonings

Stuffed bell peppers-

- ✔ Cut the top and center out of bell pepper, put standing up in vegetable steamer with taco seasoning and water cook in microwave for 7-8 minutes
- ✔ Cook 1 package 99%fat free turkey burger with taco seasoning
- ✔ Cook brown rice in rice cooker with taco seasoning
- ✔ Stuff bell peppers with turkey burger, tomatoes, rice and low fat mozzarella cheese

Turkey rice

- ✔ Cook brown rice with low sodium soy sauce
- ✔ Scramble egg whites with seasoned pepper add cut up deli turkey once eggs are cooked, cook long enough to warm turkey. Add veggies (cooked snap peas, carrots, baby corns and peas are delicious) Add little soy sauce if needed.

Chicken Rice Casserole

Put 2 cups brown rice, 4 cups frozen green beans, 16oz frozen chicken in cake pan, 2 cans enchilada sauce, season with pepper (if desired). Bake at 350 degrees for 1-4 hours (covered with tinfoil), checking every 30 minutes. Cook until rice is soft

Chicken Noodle Soup

Crock pot- add 8oz chicken, 1 cup uncooked noodles, chicken bouillon (or chicken broth), 1-2 cups frozen veggies cook until chicken is cooked and noodles soft.

CHAPTER 19

Salads and Vegetables

Cucumber salad-

- ✔ 4 lemon cucumbers, 1 regular cucumber, 20 cherry tomatoes, 1 Roma tomato, 3oz cooked chicken, 1tbsp fat free balsamic vinaigrette

Asparagus salad-

- ✔ 1-2 c lettuce
- ✔ 6 turkey pepperonis
- ✔ 4 slices deli turkey
- ✔ ¼ cup grilled asparagus- cut up asparagus put on tinfoil spray with butter flavored pam, garlic salt and parmesan cheese, wrap in foil cook on bbq grill, sprinkle parmesan cheese, salad supreme seasoning

Poppy seed chicken-

- ✔ 3-4oz grilled chicken, 1 cup lettuce, 1 cup Cole-slaw lettuce, 1 tbsp. craisins, 1 tbsp.

honey roasted peanuts or honey roasted cashews, drizzle with *Skinny Girl* poppy seed dressing (could add avocado as well)

Teriyaki bell pepper chicken-

- ✔ 3-4oz shredded chicken or canned chicken, cut bell peppers, cook on frying pan with water and 2-3 tbsp. teriyaki sauce- top of roman lettuce

Spinach strawberry salad-

- ✔ 3-4oz grilled chicken, ¼ c strawberries, 1tbsp sunflower seeds or hemp heart seeds
- ✔ ¼ avocado, 1/8c feta cheese
- ✔ Fat free raspberry vinaigrette dressing

Egg salad-

- ✔ 1-2 c Roman lettuce
- ✔ ¼ c fat free cottage cheese, 4 dill pickles, 2 hard boiled eggs (whites only), 4 slices deli turkey-cut up, seasoned pepper to taste

Grilled Asparagus-
cut up asparagus put on tinfoil spray with butter flavored pam, garlic salt and parmesan cheese, wrap in foil cook on bbq grill, sprinkle parmesan cheese, salad supreme seasoning

Cauliflower rice-
frozen cauliflower rice in vegetable steamer, add lemon pepper seasoning and water. Cook in microwave for 5-10 minutes, stir cook another 5 minutes. After this is cooked I sometimes make a teriyaki bowl with it, by adding chicken, snap peas and teriyaki sauce

Stir Fry- Snap peas, carrots in frying pan, add seasoned pepper and teriyaki sauce and water. Cook on stove, med/high with lid on stirring occasionally until the veggies are soft.

Seasoned Veggies- Mixed broccoli, cauliflower, carrots add smokey mesquite bbq seasoning and water. Cook in microwave in vegetable steamer 5-10 minutes, stir and cook another 5 minutes until soft.

Steamed Green Beans- Green beans, season with sea salt and seasoned pepper, add water and cook in vegetable steamer in microwave for 5-10 minutes, stir cook another 5.

Fresh veggies and dip- Cauliflower, broccoli, carrots, celery (cut and washed), dip in hummus.

Celery with all natural peanut butter on it.

CHAPTER 20

Other

Guacamole-

- ✔ 1 avocado mashed, 1 tomato cubed, 1/8 Italian dressing packet, squeeze lime

Peanut Butter balls-

- ✔ 1 jar *Smart Balance* peanut butter (26oz) scoop in bowl and microwave until soft
- ✔ Add 6 ½ scoops of *Muscle Pharm's* cookies n cream protein powder
- ✔ Mix those two ingredients
- ✔ Add 2 cups dried oats mix
- ✔ 1 cup frozen spinach finely chopped
- ✔ ½ craisins
- ✔ Mix- put bowl in fridge until cooled then roll into balls and stick in a freezer bag and freeze, take out as you want to snack, let thaw for about 5-10 minutes

Carrot cake balls

- 1 TBSP coconut oil
- 1/3 c almond butter
- ¼ c honey or agave nectar
- ½ c old fashioned oats
- 2 tsp. hemp hearts
- ¼ c shredded coconut
- ½ tsp cinnamon
- 1 c carrots
- Roll all together and freeze or put in fridge

Cookie dough balls

- 1 c almond flour
- 4 scoop protein (I use one of these chocolates, cookies n cream, choc Pb, vanilla)
- ½-3/4c almond milk
- ½-3/4 c Peanut Butter or almond butter
- Mix together store in fridge or freezer

Smoothie-

- 1 scoop protein, ½ c frozen spinach, 2 TBSP Peanut Butter, ½ c Greek yogurt, ½ c frozen berries, water or almond milk

Pineapple ice-cream-

- 1 chopped and frozen pineapple
- 1 ½ cups almond milk
- 1 scoop vanilla protein
- Blend

No bake cookies-

- 1cup softened smart balance Peanut Butter, 1 cup chocolate protein powder (mix together- peanut butter has to been softened in microwave first).
- Add in 1 cup of dried oats, mix, roll into balls set on a cookie sheet with tinfoil to set

Healthy nutty-butters-

- Follow above recipe for no-bake cookies. Pour in 1 cup Chex instead of oats, add ¼-½c dry roasted or dry peanuts.
- – Chocolate Chex mix
- 1 cup roasted peanuts lightly salted, 1 cup raw almonds, 1 cup raisins, 1 cup corn Chex, mix together. Take 1 scoop chocolate protein mix with a tiny bit of water, pour over Chex mix, stir up and cook on 350degrees for 20-60 minutes, checking and stirring. Cook until it's a little crisp

Trail mix-

- 1c of all- natural almonds, cashews with sea salt, favas peas sea salt, dry roasted peanuts lightly salted, raisins
- 2 cups- craisins
- ½-1 c *Pascha 85%* cacao dark chocolate chips

Banana oatmeal cookies-

- 3 mashed bananas (ripe)
- 1/3 c apple sauce

- ✔ 2 cups oats
- ✔ ¼ c almond milk
- ✔ 1 tsp vanilla
- ✔ 1 tsp cinnamon
- ✔ Bake at 350 for 15-20 minutes.

Chocolate fudge-

- ✔ Bottom layer-
- ✔ ½ c smart balance Peanut Butter
- ✔ 1/3 c almond butter
- ✔ ½ tbsp. vanilla
- ✔ ½ tbsp. agave nectar
- ✔ (Mix above- lay flat in a small cake dish)
- ✔ Top layer-
- ✔ ½ c Peanut Butter
- ✔ 1/3c almond milk
- ✔ 1 scoop chocolate protein powder
- ✔ 1 tbsp. agave nectar
- ✔ Add water if it's too thick- to make consistency of brownie batter
- ✔ Spread on top of bottom layer
- ✔ Put in fridge for 2-4 hours (keep in fridge)

Chocolate banana bread-

- ✔ Mix in medium bowl-
- ✔ 5 very ripe bananas (mashed and mix with beaters) then add other ingredients
- ✔ 1 1 /2 c almond flour
- ✔ 1 tsp of baking soda
- ✔ 1 egg white
- ✔ 2 TBSP stevia sugar replacement
- ✔ Sprinkle cinnamon

- ✔ Mix again
- ✔ Add 10-20 semi sweet choc chips (or dark chocolate chips)
- ✔ Bake at 325 for 40 minutes

Fruit dip-

- ✔ Mix any flavor of single serving *Dannon Fit* and Light Greek yogurt with ¼c cottage cheese or ¼c cream cheese if you don't like cottage cheese

Berry ice-cream-

- ✔ 1 ½ single serving *Dannon Greek* yogurt strawberry cheesecake
- ✔ 1 cup frozen strawberries, blueberries and raspberries
- ✔ ½ c almond milk
- ✔ Mix with beaters- serve

Berry PB ice-cream-

- ✔ Same as above add 1 tbsp. smart balance Peanut Butter

Chocolate Peanut Butter ice-cream-

- ✔ 1 *Dannon* Greek yogurt coconut vanilla, 1 ½ frozen bananas, 1 scoop chocolate protein, 1 tbsp. Peanut Butter, ½ c almond milk mix with blender

Cottage cheese/ yogurt

- ✔ ½ cup cottage cheese and ½ c flavored yogurt mix together. Can also add frozen grapes or other frozen fruit to this

CHAPTER 21

Grocery lists

Costco grocery List-

Frozen-

- ✔ *Kirkland's* chicken tenders
- ✔ Frozen mixed veggies
- ✔ Frozen green beans
- ✔ Frozen peas
- ✔ Frozen berries
- ✔ Frozen mangoes

FRESH-

- ✔ Hearts of roman lettuce (pack of 6)
- ✔ Raspberries
- ✔ Blackberries
- ✔ Sweet potatoes
- ✔ Sugar snap peas
- ✔ Small carrots
- ✔ Liquid egg whites

GROCERY-

- *Quaker* old fashioned oats
- *Kids Cliff* Z bars
- *Nature valley* bars
- Craisins
- Organic millet and brown rice Ramon noodles
- *Kirkland* canned chicken
- *McCormick* taco seasoning
- Teriyaki sauce
- *Kirkland* canned green beans
- *Kirkland* canned tomato sauce
- *Kodiak Cake* buttermilk pancake mix
- *Kodiak Cake* berry syrup

<u>Grocery store-</u>

Produce-

- Tomatoes (if it's off season and I don't have them in the garden)
- Apples
- Bananas
- Grapes (red ones are delicious to freeze)
- Avocado
- Red potatoes

Grocery-

- 99%fat free ground turkey
- Low fat turkey pepperonis
- Low fat mozzarella cheese
- *Dannon Fit* and Light Greek yogurt
- Unsweetened vanilla almond milk
- Rice cakes (chocolate, caramel, and mini

cheese, ranch)
- ✔ *Smart Balance* Peanut butter
- ✔ *Smuckers low sugar jelly*
- ✔ *Skinny girl* salad dressing
- ✔ BBQ sauce
- ✔ Fat Free Italian dressing
- ✔ Alfredo packets, pesto packets, (cook with water instead of oil)
- ✔ *Pita flatbread*
- ✔ *Missions whole wheat tortillas*
- ✔ Whole wheat noodles

Couscous

- ✔ *Amazing Grass* green superfood antioxidant sweet berry (can also be found at *Amazon*)

Seasonings-

- ✔ *Lawry's-* seasoned pepper, garlic pepper, lemon pepper, garlic salt
- ✔ *Weber-* Smokey mesquite
- ✔ *McCormick's-* salad supreme, sweet & Smokey, mesquite rub,
- ✔ *Wyler's* chicken bouillon cubes

Cinnamon-

I hope you have enjoyed this super easy way to understand food and proper nutrition. I had so much fun digging up some of these old recipes that I love! I hope you will use this guide as a way to make healthier food choices for you and your family! If you have questions or need help beyond this book, please email me, Amara@TeamCrazyFit.com I offer personalized meal plans, workout plans, personal training, macro counts and more. I truly love teaching others how to live a healthier lifestyle, and I truly hope this book has helped you have a better understanding of food!

I invite you to follow me on Instagram- **TeamCrazyFit** and on Facebook- **Team Crazy Fit**, where I post my latest recipes, fitness tips and workouts.

Happy Health to You!

www.ingramcontent.com/pod-product-compliance
Lightning Source LLC
Chambersburg PA
CBHW062149020426
42334CB00020B/2553